The Power of Breathing Techniques

Breathing Exercises for more Fitness, Health and Relaxation

©2019, Lutz Schneider

Published by Expertengruppe

D1528006

The Power of Breathing Techniques

Breathing Exercises for more Fitness, Health and Relaxation

Published by Expertengruppe

TABLE OF CONTENTS

About the author

Lutz Schneider lives with his wife, Doris, in an old farmhouse in beautiful Rhineland.

Ever since he studied the biology of evolution, over 20 years ago, he has been interested in marginal health subjects, which are often hidden from the main stream, but which are scientifically well accepted. He teaches this knowledge, not only to his students, but also reaches a wider audience in Germany with his various publications.

In his books, he speaks about subjects, the positive effects of which are widely unknown and on which he can pass on his own experiences. All of his publications, therefore, are based on indisputable scientific facts, but also encompass his own very personal experiences and knowledge. This way, the reader not only receives factual information about the subject but also a practical guide with a wide range of knowledge and useful tips, which are easy to understand and put into practice.

Lutz Schneider's easy to read work puts the reader into a relaxed and pleasant ambience, while gaining insight into a subject which few know anything about but which everyone could profit from.

Preface

Congratulations, you have made an excellent decision to take care of your fitness, health and recreation needs. In addition, you have decided to buy this guide, so you have already made two good choices.

We can survive for weeks without food and days without water, but only a few minutes without air. While we think a lot about what we eat and drink, we do not really care much about the air that we breathe. It is generally known that our daily consumption of nourishment and water has to abide by quality and quantity standards. Too much or too little will cause problems. We also know the importance of breathing good quality air, but how much is good? How much air should we breathe for optimum health? Would it not be justified to presume that the air, which is more important for human survival than food or water, should live up to basic standards? The amount of air that you breathe has the potential to change everything you believe about your body, your health and your performance. This is true, whether you are an active person, someone who rarely gets off the couch, a recreational sportsman, who sometimes runs 10 miles, or a professional athlete who needs a decisive advantage over his competition.

Perhaps you are asking yourself what I mean with amount. After all, air is not something you can nibble on at the kitchen table or drink too much of at the weekend. But what if, in a certain way, it was like that? What if healthy breathing habits were as important, if not more so, than good nutrition, in order to attain maximum fitness and health?

In this book, you will discover the fundamental relationship between Oxygen and your body. The improvement of your fitness depends on the release of Oxygen and your muscles, organs and tissue. Increasing your Oxygen supply is not only healthy, it enables an increase in the intensity of your training and also reduces breathlessness. In short, you will notice an improvement in your health, and more relaxation in your everyday life.

If you take part in competitions, you will enjoy your training and your competitive events more than ever, because you will be able to achieve more. Generally, fitness and sport performance are limited by your lungs - not by your legs, arms or even your mind. Everyone who regularly does sport knows that the feeling of being out of breath influences the intensity of your training much more than the tiredness of your muscles. The basis for health and the improvement of physical activity, therefore, has to involve optimising respiratory function.

Are you ready to invest time and willpower into the optimisation of your breathing technique?

Then you have made the right choice and are ready to read the following pages!

From my heart, I wish you much success and good luck.

The Secret of Oxygen

Your Respiratory System

Before you begin with the breathing exercises, it is important that you learn the fundamentals of the breathing organs and the role which Carbon Dioxide and Nitrogen Oxide have in your body. The more you know, the more you will be able to work with your body instead of against it.

Your respiratory system encompasses the parts of your body which release Oxygen into your cells and transport the Carbon Dioxide, which is produced in the tissue, back out into the atmosphere. Your respiratory system contains everything you need to provide your body with enough Oxygen to carry out sports, including high-performance sports, as long as you allow it to function properly.

When we breathe, air flows into the body and down the windpipe (trachea), which in turn divides into two branches which are called the bronchi: One branch leads to the left lung and the other to the right lung. Inside the lungs, the bronchi divide further into smaller branches, or twigs, which are called bronchioles, and eventually into a myriad of air sacks which are called alveoli. In order to visualise this complex system, imagine an upside-down tree.

Your windpipe is the trunk of the tree and the bronchi are the larger branches, from which the twigs of the bronchioles are growing. At the end of these twigs are the "leaves", the round bags known as the alveoli, which transport the Oxygen into the blood. It is an impressive example of evolutionary balance and beauty, that the trees around us, which release Oxygen, have a similar structure to the lungs that receive it.

The body has about 300 million alveoli which are surrounded by tiny blood vessels called capillaries. To get the enormous numbers into perspective, the contact surface area between your alveoli and your blood capillaries would cover a tennis court. This huge, impressive surface area has the potential to form an extremely efficient Oxygen transmission system into the blood.

As I already explained, Oxygen is the fuel that the muscles need to work efficiently. It is a common mistake to believe that breathing in a greater volume of air would lead to an increased supply of Oxygen in the blood. It is physiologically impossible to increase the Oxygen saturation of the blood in this way, because the blood is almost always fully saturated. It would be like pouring water into a glass which is already full to the brim.

What is Oxygen saturation, exactly, and how does it connect to the correct Oxygen supply in the muscles?

Oxygen saturation (SpO2) is the percentage of Oxygen-carrying red blood corpuscles (haemoglobin molecules), which are present in the blood. During rest periods, the standard breathing volume for a healthy person amounts to between 1 and 1.6 gallons of air per minute. This represents an almost complete Oxygen saturation of between 95 and 99 percent. As Oxygen continually diffuses from the blood into the cells, a 100 percent saturation is not always possible. An Oxygen saturation of 100 percent would suggest that the link between the red corpuscles and the Oxygen molecules is too strong, which would diminish the ability of the blood corpuscles to release Oxygen to the muscles, organs and tissue.

We need the blood to release the Oxygen, not to retain it. The human body carries a surplus of Oxygen in the blood. About 75 percent of the Oxygen is breathed out, unused, during rest periods, and even up to 25 percent during physical exertion. The increase in Oxygen saturation to 100 percent, therefore, will not serve any useful purpose.

The idea that taking larger breaths would increase your Oxygen intake is like telling someone, who already eats enough to cover his daily calorie requirements, that he must eat more. Many people have difficulty with this concept. They have been "taught" about the advantages of deep breathing for years by stress management advisors, yoga practitioners, physiotherapists and sport trainers, let alone from the Western media.

It is easy to understand why this belief is perpetuated: Taking a deep breath can really make you feel good, even if it is not really good for you. Similar to a cat having a good stretch after his afternoon nap, deep breaths into the lungs stretch the upper body so that you feel more relaxed. This, however, leads to the assumption that "bigger" also means "better".

Regulating your Respiration

There are two main aspects regarding the way you breathe:

1. The frequency or number of breaths you take in a minute

2. The volume or amount of air which flows into the lungs with each breath.

Even though they are different, one generally influences the other. The volume of every breath, in and out, is measured in litres and the measurement is normally carried out over a period of exactly one minute.

In general medicine, it is considered that a healthy person would breathe 10 to 12 times with every breath being about 0.13 gallons, making a total volume of 1.3 or 1.6 gallons of air per minute. To help you visualise this amount of air, imagine how much air would fit into one and a half gallon packs of milk. If someone breathes at a higher frequency, for example at 20 breaths per minute, logically the volume would increase. Over-breathing not only happens when someone breathes too quickly, a lower breathing speed can also have the same effect if, for example, the person breathes 10 times, each breath being a litre in volume.

You will find out why over-breathing is harmful in the following pages.

Carbon Dioxide as the metronome of your Respiration

How CO2 Controls your Breathing

How can we ensure optimum use of our astonishing breathing apparatus, using breathing techniques? As strange as it may seem, it is not the Oxygen which has the primary influence on our respiratory function but the Carbon Dioxide (CO2). Your breathing frequency and volume are regulated by receptors in the brain which work like the thermostat of a heating system in a house.

Instead of controlling the temperature variation, these receptors regulate the concentration of Carbon Dioxide and Oxygen in the blood as well as the acidic or pH value. When the amount of Carbon Dioxide rises over a specific volume, these sensitive receptors stimulate the respiration to remove the excess gas. In other words, the primary stimulus to breathe is to remove excess Carbon Dioxide from the body.

Carbon Dioxide is the end product of a natural process of reducing the fat and Carbohydrates which we take into our bodies. The CO2 drains out of the tissue through the blood vessels and cells into the lungs and the surplus is exhaled. It is crucial that some of the Carbon Dioxide is retained in the body after exhaling. Correct breathing is the prerequisite so that the right amount of Carbon Dioxide remains in the lungs. It is just as important for everyone to understand this, whether you are an ambitious sportsman or just interested in basic fitness or losing weight. The correct amount of Carbon Dioxide in the body has an equal role to play in influencing your immune system and your psychological condition. The body can only work quietly and maintain relaxation when it has stored the correct amount of Carbon Dioxide. Every time the body is subject to over- or undersaturation, it becomes stressed. This can also take the form of mental stress.

Imagine it like this: The CO_2 is the door through which the Oxygen passes into our muscles. If the door is only partly open, only part of our available Oxygen can pass through it, so that we begin to pant and our limbs start to cramp. If, on the other hand, the door is open widely, a large amount of Oxygen can flow through it and we can continue our physical activities longer and with a higher intensity. However, in order to understand how our respiration works, we have to look closer at the decisive role that Carbon Dioxide plays in maximising efficiency.

Chronic hyperventilation or over-breathing is the habit of breathing in more air than the body needs. It does not always manifest itself as a dramatic symptom, like someone gasping during a panic attack. If we breathe more than necessary, too much Carbon Dioxide is released out of the lungs and is therefore removed from the blood. It forces the door into the closed position, so that it becomes more difficult to allow Oxygen to pass.

Breathing too deeply over a short period of time is not a great problem and does not cause any long-term changes in the body. However, if we breathe too deeply over a period of several days, a biological change happens in our bodies, leading to increased sensitivity or tolerance to Carbon Dioxide. In this case, the respiratory volume remains above the normal amount because the receptors in the brain are continually stimulating the respiration in order to get rid of the volume of Carbon Dioxide, which the receptor accepts as its normal value.

This results in the bad habit of chronic over-breathing with all its negative manifestations. In other words: Under certain circumstances, our body gets used to breathing in a way that is against its own interests. In order to counteract this, you need to form better breathing habits.

Here, I would like to mention an important point: As you have learned, correct respiration has an enormous influence on our health. You should pay particular attention to carrying out the exercises in this book correctly. Incorrect or bad breathing techniques can have dramatic health, psycho-logical and physical consequences.

The volume of a breath could be two or three times greater than necessary, without being obviously noticeable. Once the pattern of over-breathing has become established, this will often be sustained by taking a deep breath or sigh. If this habit becomes anchored, you will be breathing more than you need each minute, each hour and each day. This subtle change in the natural function of your body can cause a lot of harm.

This happens not only while we are awake, many people sleep with open mouths and, whether they know it or not, this reduces your physical and mental energy. Why are the advantages of light breathing relatively unknown? It is difficult to find the exact answer to that, although we should take a series of facts into consideration.

Firstly, air is weightless and therefore difficult to measure. Respiration could change during the measuring process quickly and unnoticed. In addition, doctors learn early in their studies that Oxygen is released out of the red corpuscles, so if this information comes at the end of their studies, it could easily be forgotten.

A further reason could be that hyperventilation can cause different, seemingly unconnected, problems in different people – from cardio-vascular, respiratory and gastrointestinal problems or perhaps to general exhaustion. To cause even more confusion, not everyone who over-breathes, suffers from obvious symptoms as the impact of the hyperventilation is also dependent upon genetic predisposition.

Given the lack of awareness of the connection between breathing volume and health, many chronic over-breathers have learned to tolerate the stunted energy level and lack of fitness which has been caused by constant incorrect breathing.

However, if we manage to shake ourselves out of our complacency regarding respiration and start to make this the centre of our health regime, dramatic results can occur, such as those you would notice after dietary change. How can we regulate the amount of air we breathe in order to optimise our fitness and sport performance? As you already know, the main component is Carbon Dioxide.

CO2: Not only bad air

The natural Carbon Dioxide concentration in the Earth's atmosphere is very low. This means that we transport very little Carbon Dioxide into our lungs when breathing. Instead we produce our own CO_2 in the cells of our tissue, during the process of converting food and Oxygen into energy. The correct breathing volume is dependent upon our ability to maintain an ideal amount of Carbon Dioxide in the lungs, blood, tissue and cells.

Carbon Dioxide fulfils important functions in the human body, including:

- The discharge of Oxygen from the blood, which is needed by the cells.

- The stretching of the smooth muscles in the walls of the breathing apparatus and blood vessels.

- The regulation of the blood's PH value.

The Bohr Effect

Haemoglobin is a protein which Is present in the blood. Its function is to transport Oxygen from the lungs to the tissues and cells. One of the main elements of the breathing techniques in this book is the understanding of the Bohr Effect – the way in which Oxygen is released from the Haemoglobin into the muscles and organs. This process forms the core of developing the fitness potential of your body, so that you can increase your performance and obtain the results that you really want.

The Bohr Effect was discovered in 1904 by the Danish Physiologist, Christian Bohr (the father of Niels Bohr, Nobel Prize winner in Physics). Christian Bohr: "The Carbon Dioxide pressure in the blood can be seen as an important factor in the metabolism of the inner breathing passages. If the appropriate amount of Carbon Dioxide is used, the Oxygen present in the whole body can be better used." Most importantly, Oxygen is released when Haemoglobin and Carbon Dioxide are present.

When we over-breathe, too much Carbon Dioxide is washed out of the lungs, blood, tissue and cells. This condition is called Hypocapnia. This causes the Haemoglobin to retain Oxygen, which, in turn, leads to a reduction in the supply of Oxygen to the tissue and organs. When the muscles receive less Oxygen, they cannot work as effectively as we would wish them to. So, as counter-intuitive as it may seem, the urge to take deeper breaths, when you have reached your limit during training, does not increase the supply of Oxygen to your muscles, but reduces the intake of Oxygen even more.

On the contrary, the Carbon Dioxide pressure in the blood is higher when the breathing volume remains closer to the optimum level. The bond between Haemoglobin and Oxygen loosens and the Oxygen supply can more easily reach the muscles and organs. A trained muscle is hot, caused by Carbon Dioxide and it profits from an increased discharge of O2 (Oxygen) from the capillaries. The more we supply our muscles with Oxygen during activity, the longer and harder they can work. With respect to the Bohr Effect, over-breathing limits the release of Oxygen out of the blood and this, in turn, influences how well our muscles work.

Enlargement and Narrowing of the Respiratory Tract and Blood Vessels

Breathing too heavily can also lead to reduced blood flow. For the majority of people, two minutes of heavy breathing can lead to a reduction of the flood flow throughout the body, including the brain. This can lead to a feeling of dizziness and drowsiness. Generally, the reduction in blood flow to the brain is proportional to each reduction in Carbon Dioxide.

Most people have already experienced a narrowing of the blood flow to the brain through over-breathing. It only takes a short while, taking large breaths in and out through the mouth, before dizziness can be felt. In addition, it can be difficult for those people, who sleep with their mouths open, to get moving in the mornings. No matter how long they have slept, during the first couple of hours after waking up, they will feel tired and groggy.

Various studies have concluded that people who usually breathe through their mouths during waking and sleeping hours, suffer from tiredness, lack of concentration, reduced productivity and bad moods, not really an ideal recipe for quality of life or a productive training programme.

The same can be said for people whose work entails long periods of speaking, for example, a teacher or sales representative. People in these professions are only too aware of how tired they are after a day's work – but the exhaustion after endless meetings is not necessarily due to mental or physical exertion, but due to the increase in breathing rate during that time. It is normal for the breathing rate to increase during physical exertion because the body needs more

Oxygen, in order to convert food into energy. While speaking, the breathing rate increases, even though no extra Oxygen is needed. This leads to a disturbance of blood gases and a reduction of the blood flow.

If you are genetically prone to asthma, the loss of Carbon Dioxide in the blood can lead the smooth muscles of the respiratory system to narrow, which in turn can lead to panting and breathlessness. However, an increase in Carbon Dioxide can open these airways and improve the transport of Oxygen and it has become apparent that the respiration of people with asthma also improves. At the end of the day we move between both sides of the spectrum; of good breathing on one side and bad breathing on the other. It is not only people with asthma who can profit from less narrow airways.

That feeling of tightness in the chest, excessive breathlessness, coughing and inability to take a fulfilling breath is recognisable to every athlete, including those who have no history of asthma. This, however, be remedied by simply improving the respiratory function.

Regulating the Blood PH Values

In addition to the provision of Oxygen to the tissue and cells, Carbon Dioxide also plays a central role in regulating the PH value in the bloodstream. It regulates how acidic or alkaline your blood is. The normal PH value in the blood is about 7.365 and this value needs to be kept around that number to prevent the body forcing some kind of compensatory measures. If, for example, the PH value in the blood increases its alkaline value, respiration slows, so that the level of Carbon Dioxide increases to restore the PH value back to normal. Because Carbon Dioxide is an acid, an increase in the amount of Carbon Dioxide in the blood will reverse the process.

If the PH value of the blood is too acidic (from, for example, an excess in consumption of processed foods) the breathing rate increases to release the Carbon Dioxide at a higher rate in order to reduce the acid to normal levels. Sustaining a normal PH value in the blood is essential for our survival. When the PH value is too acidic, and falls below 6.8, or becomes too alkaline and rises above 7.8, the result can be fatal. The reason for this is that the PH value directly influences the functionality of our inner organs and metabolism.

Scientific findings show clearly that Carbon Dioxide is a major element which not only regulates breathing, optimises the blood flow and transports Oxygen to the muscles, but also ensures the correct PH value. In short, the relationship of Carbon Dioxide with our bodies determines how healthy we can be and influences almost every aspect of the body's function. Through better respiration, Carbon Dioxide ensures that the inter-connected parts of our system work harmoniously with each other, so that we can exploit our maximum potential in sporting performance, endurance and strength.

Without the required amount of CO_2 in the blood the blood vessels are restricted and the Haemoglobin can not transport Oxygen into the bloodstream. Without the required amount of Oxygen, the muscles cannot function as effectively as they should. We become breathless or reach the limits of our abilities. It becomes a cycle: It is not only breathless exertion that lead to panting. It is the panting which leads to breathless exertion.

In the following chapters, you will learn how you can break this cycle and establish a new, positive cycle. The elimination of over-breathing is the key to utilising the potential of the Carbon Dioxide that you already have inside you. The first step in the empowerment process is to understand how respiration works.

*A brief conclusion: Breathing more and with it, increasing the Oxygen intake, is not automatically better! Both too much and too little Oxygen can be damaging to you! To stay fit, healthy and relaxed, you must train your body to absorb the **optimum** amount of Oxygen.*

Breathing through the nose is the key to success

The Advantages of Nose-breathing compared to Mouth-breathing

In order to learn the correct breathing technique, the first step is to return to the basics and learn to breathe through the nose, day and night. Every child knows that the nose is for breathing and the mouth for eating. You were born, breathing through the nose and it has always been the body's main passage for respiration. It was only when our oldest ancestors found themselves in the most dangerous situations that they changed to mouth-breathing in order to take in larger amounts of air as preparation for a fight for life or death.

For this reason, breathing through the mouth is synonymous with a total emergency situation which, with our ancestors, activated a fight-or-flight reaction. Today, it is not accompanied by any physical effort which would cause the body's own operating system to normalise itself. Respiratory physiology shows that breathing through the mouth activates the upper chest, whereas breathing through the mouth activates abdominal respiration. You can check the difference by sitting in front of a mirror, one hand on your chest and one hand over your naval.

When you have settled down, take a medium-sized breath through the mouth and notice the movement under your hands. Next compare the movement after breathing a similar amount of air through the nose. The movement of the upper chest is connected more with a stress reaction, whereas nose breathing ensures peaceful and even breathing, extending the diaphragm.

The popular misconception of breathing "deeply" is to "blow up" the chest and raise the shoulders, but this is neither deep, nor advantageous for the Oxygen supply of the body. In order to cope with stress, this is essentially correct, but a really deep breath comes from the abdomen and is gentle and peaceful; the exact opposite to the big breaths that would normally be taken to try and bring about a calm state.

Breathing through the mouth activates the chest. You take larger breaths and this can cause a decrease in Oxygen in the arterial blood. It is no surprise that people who usually breathe through their mouths often lack energy, have poor concentration and suffer from mood swings. If you think I am being overly critical, I

was a mouth-breather for more than 15 years –
this is how I know the consequences only too
well.

Apart from that, I see the result of long-term
mouth-breathing when I look in the mirror.
Dentists and orthodontists have documented
the profound facial changes caused by mouth-
breathing: narrower jaw, crooked teeth, sunken
cheekbones and smaller nostrils. While
orthodontic treatment and the wearing of braces
is an epidemic with today's youth, it was normal
for our ancestors to have full faces with perfectly
formed teeth.

Nose-breathing is often an essential part of the
survival or hunting technique of animals. The
cheetah, who is known as the fastest land animal
in the world, is able to accelerate from 0 to 100
kilometres per hour in only 3 seconds. Most high-
performance cars are not able to keep pace with

that. With such efficiency and speed, it does not take long for the cheetah to catch up with its prey. Nose-breathing is particularly advantageous during the hunt because it ensures that the predator's victim runs out of breath first.

The dog is probably the best-known example of an animal which regularly breathes through its mouth. You often see how it pants, to cool itself off, on a hot day or after a long walk. However, in all other cases the dog breathes through its nose and uses its mouth to eat, drink and bark. Mother Nature has made sure that the large majority of land mammals breathe through their noses by positioning the airpipe so that the bridge of the nose leads directly into the lungs. In other words, it is not easy for most animals to breathe through the mouth.

The same applies to humans when they are born. After a few months, the airpipe sinks to just above the back of the tongue, so that a baby can breathe both through its nose and mouth. Charles Darwin was confused by this adaptation. With humans, the openings for the transport of food into the stomach and air into the lungs, are placed side by side, contrary to almost all animals. This parallel position does not seem very practical as it increases the risk of food passing in the wrong direction, which in turn requires a complicated mechanism for swallowing.

The origin of this adaptation lies probably with our ability to speak and swim. Both of these activities require voluntary control over the breathing. If Darwin had investigated the negative effects of mouth-breathing in humans, I have no doubt that he would have found that the ability to mouth-breathe is a much worse mistake in evolution than the risk of choking while eating.

The rest of the animal world relies on nose-breathing for its survival. Mouth-breathing is mostly a result of adaptation of a particular species to its lifestyle. Birds, for example, are mostly nose-breathers, apart from those who dive, like penguins, pelicans or gannets, which breathe through their mouths. Generally, breathing through the mouth is a sign of sickness, injury or distress.

Guinea-pigs and rabbits continue to breathe through the nose, even during strenuous periods and breathe only through the mouth when they have some kind of disorder. The same applies to livestock, including cows, sheep, donkeys, goats and horses. The mouth-breathing of these animals is a clear signal to the farmer or pet owner that something is wrong. Practice has shown the farmer that it is time to call the vet when a cow or sheep is standing, motionless, with a stretched neck and open mouth.

In order to get an idea of the size of the nasal cavity, allow your tongue to go back from the front of the gums to the back as far as it can. You will be surprised when you realise that your gum is actually the nasal floor! The nose that you see in your face is only about 30% of its total volume. You could say it is the tip of the iceberg. The other 70% of the nasal cavity lies deep inside the skull. Mother Nature is intelligent and wastes no space; evolution has determined how much space your nose deserves to take up inside your skull.

When air streams through the nose, it is forced through a curved, spongy bone, the so-called concha. The inhaled air is then swirled around and conditioned into an even, regular mass. The inner nose, with its dead-ends, valves and the concha regulate the direction and speed of the air in order to maximise its influence through a net of small arteries, veins and the mucus membrane; to warm the air; to moisturise and sterilise it, before it enters the lungs.

Functions of Nose-breathing

Below you will find a short list of the functions of nose-breathing:

- In normal people, nose-breathing creates approximately 50% more resistance to the airflow than mouth-breathing, which leads to an increase of between 10 and 20 percent in O2 intake.

- Nose-breathing warms and moisturises the incoming air. Air, which is breathed in at a temperature of 43°F, is warmed to approximately 86°F by the time it reaches the back of the throat and is at a comfortable 99°F when it reaches its final destination – the lungs.

- Nose-breathing removes a large number of germs and bacteria from the air that you breathe in. Breathing through the mouth causes a higher number of germs to reach the lungs and from there possibly also into the bloodstream.

- During physical exercise, nose-breathing enables a work intensity which is high enough to create an aerobic effect, based on the heart frequency and a higher intake of Oxygen.

- As will be mentioned in the next section, the nose is a reservoir for Nitrogen Oxide, an essential gas for the maintenance of health.

Compare the above-mentioned advantages with the effects of mouth-breathing:

- Children who breathe through their mouths have an increased risk of developing a posture where the head is leaning forward and breathing power is reduced.

- Breathing through the mouth can lead to general dehydration (mouth-breathing during sleep leads to waking up with a dry mouth).

- A dry mouth can increase oral acidification and can lead to more tooth decay and gum disease.

- Mouth-breathing can cause bad breath due to altered bacterial flora.

- Mouth-breathing significantly increases the instances of snoring and sleep apnoea.

Another short conclusion: The worst mistake most people make is frequent, subconscious mouth-breathing. The disadvantages of mouth-breathing are immense! Nose-breathing is the natural and optimum way to provide the body with Oxygen and keep it healthy and fit!

Nose-breathing at Night

The ideal amount of sleep a body needs varies from person to person. The late British Prime Minister, Margaret Thatcher, is said to have only needed four hours sleep, but most of us need seven or eight hours of good sleep to make us fit for the next day. If we have difficulty in going to sleep, or if the sleep is disturbed through snoring or sleep apnoea, it can be very difficult to get up the following morning and can significantly affect performance, concentration, mood and even the most basic of activities.

Even when we seem to sleep through the night, the quality of our sleep can be adversely affected, so that we have a dry mouth and a feeling of listlessness when we wake up. All you need to do is to close your mouth while you are sleeping. If you would not like to use tape at night, a chin strap would be a good alternative and would help prevent the lower jaw from falling during sleep.

Chin straps are often used by people with obstructive sleep apnoea and can be bought easily through the internet. Immobilising the mouth at night also ensures that you can breathe well while sleeping, you can fall asleep quicker and sleep longer, so that you feel energised when you wake up. If you often wake up with a dry mouth in the morning it is a sign that you have been breathing through the mouth. In that case, you should consider obtaining a chin strap. Your health and body will thank you for it.

The Secret of Nitrogen Oxide

Up to the 1980s, Nitrogen Monoxide (NO) was regarded as a poisonous gas which caused smog and other harmful impacts on the environment. When the first articles appeared, discussing the importance of Nitrogen Monoxide, it was difficult for the scientists to believe that a gas which was so poisonous outside of the body could have such an important role inside the body. Although Nitrogen Monoxide is a relative newcomer to the area of medicine, there are now over a hundred-thousand research projects involving this gas, giving a clue as to how doctors and scientists have now focused their attention on this subject.

In 1992 Nitrogen Monoxide was declared "molecule of the year" by the publication "Science". It was described as an amazingly simple molecule that unites neuroscience, physiology and immunology and which has revised the opinions of scientists regarding their understanding of how cells communicate and defend themselves.

In 1998, Robert F. Furchgott, Louis J Ignarro and Ferid Murad received the Nobel Prize for their discovery that Nitrogen Monoxide is an important signal molecule within the cardiovascular system. When I was just starting to understand the advantages of Nitrogen Monoxide, I was amazed how a simple gas could influence all the important systems and organs, keep us free from diseases, like Cancer, and promote longer life. There is even proof of the positive effect of Nitrogen Monoxide on the sexual organs, a subject which we will cover later.

Curiously, it seems that, despite its life-changing properties, few people outside of medicine know the enormous health advantages of this gas. Of the hundreds of people I have spoken to, who suffer from high blood pressure, bad cardiovascular health, asthma and other sicknesses, none of them were aware of the importance of Nitrogen Monoxide.

During nose-breathing and breath-holding exercises, Nitrogen Monoxide plays an important role. Nitrogen Monoxide is produced inside the nasal cavity and the inside surfaces of the thousands of kilometres of blood vessels throughout the body.

Scientific findings show that this unusual molecule is released into the nasal airways and is transferred to the lower airways and the lungs through nose-breathing. In the prestigious journal, Thorax, the researchers Jon Lundberg and Eddie Weitzberg, from the famous Karolinska Institut in Sweden, reported that

Nitrogen Monoxide (NO) is released into the nasal airways of humans and that, while breathing through the nose, the NO follows the airstream into the lower airways and the lungs.

In view of the importance that the role which Nitrogen Monoxide plays in the provision of Oxygen to the body, Dr Mehmet Oz recommends diaphragm-respiration, because it brings Nitrogen Monoxide from the back of the nose and sinuses into the lungs. This short-lived gas extends the airways into the lungs and equally into the blood vessels. Nose-breathing is essential in using the advantages of Nitrogen Monoxide, working together with abdominal breathing, in order to maximise the Oxygen supply to the body.

Think of the nose as a reservoir: Every time we breathe softly and slowly through the nose, we are allowing this powerful molecule to enter the lungs and the blood, where it can carry out its work throughout the body. Mouth-breathing bypasses this special gas and disregards the important advantages of Nitrogen Monoxide to the general well-being of the body.

Nitrogen Monoxide plays an important role in:

- Vessel regulation: Regulating the blood vessels by opening and shutting them.

- Homeostasis: The way our body maintains a stable physiological balance in order to ensure survival.

- Neurotransmission: The messaging system in the brain.

- Immune defence: Respiration

It helps to prevent high blood pressure, reduces the cholesterol levels, keeps the arteries young and flexible and prevents blockages of the arteries through plaque and clotting. All these advantages reduce the risk of heart attacks and strokes, two of the most frequent causes of death in Germany.

With increasing age, our blood vessels lose their flexibility and the circulation reduces throughout the body. It is no coincidence that, the older a man becomes, the more apparent the signs of decreasing blood circulation become, including the occurrence of erectile dysfunction. The effectiveness of Nitrogen Monoxide in opening the blood vessels becomes clear if you consider that this simple gas plays such an important role in the erection of the penis. This discovery in 1998 led to the production of Viagra, a very popular medicine which has enjoyed many thousands of hours of media transmission time and made many millions of Euros in turnover for its manufacturer, Pfizer.

There are many reasons for breathing through the mouth, including swelling of the tissue in the nose and the formation of polyps. In a study with a group of 33 men with nose polyps, the researchers discovered that erectile dysfunction in this group was much higher. Once the men were operated on to remove the polyps, restoring nose-breathing, their erectile dysfunction became significantly reduced.

Women can also benefit from Nitrogen Monoxide as it plays a similar role in the female genitalia and increases libido. Is it possible that nose-breathers have more sexual desire and a better sex life than mouth-breathers? In addition to the improvement in sex life, this unique gas works as a defence system against micro-organisms because of its anti-viral and antibacterial effects, reducing the risk of sickness and generally improving health.

Nitrogen Monoxide plays a particularly important role with sportsmen, who want to optimise their performance, by expanding the smooth muscle layer which is embedded in the airways. Open airways enable better transfer of Oxygen from and to the lungs during training, whereas tight airways cause discomfort and inefficiency and lead to poorer performance.

How to Increase Production of Nitrogen Monoxide

The production of Nitrogen Monoxide in the sinuses can be increased by simply humming. In an article which appeared in a well-known medical journal, the doctors Weitzberg and Lundberg describe how humming increases the Nitrogen Monoxide fifteen times over compared to peaceful breathing out. They came to the conclusion that humming dramatically increases the intake of breath into the sinuses and the release of nasal Nitrogen Monoxide.

With this knowledge, it is no wonder that humming is also practised in certain meditation techniques. The breathing technique called Brahmari includes taking slow and deep breaths through the nose, while every exhalation is accompanied by a hum similar to that which a bee makes. Even though the exact science was probably unknown to him, the creator of the technique would have noticed that the feelings associated with it were beneficial.

Another short conclusion: Nitrogen Monoxide (NO) is a little miracle cure in the human body. Not much is known about the positive effect of NO, generally. Despite that, the science is documented and indisputable. The most effective method of optimising the Nitrogen Monoxide in your body is to breathe correctly. This works best using consistent nose-breathing.

Exercise No 1: Freeing the Nose

This first exercise helps mouth breathers to relax the nose and to enable consistent nose-breathing. Further breathing exercises will follow to help you find the optimum breathing technique.

Mouth-breathing causes inflammation and enlargement of the blood vessels in the nose. The increase in mucous secretion gives the feeling of nasal congestion. If the nose is blocked it is much more difficult to breathe through it, which in turn perpetuates the mouth-breathing. Continued mouth-breathing leads to a permanent condition of nasal congestion and closes the vicious cycle.

Obstructions in the nose are one of the most common symptoms of Rhinitis, which affects many people throughout the whole Western world. The main treatments for this include avoiding the origins (for example pollen) and the use of decongestants, cortisone nose sprays, anti-histamines or allergy injections. Although these treatments can alleviate the symptoms, they only work as long as you take them.

The following is a wonderful exercise to relax your nose. (Please do not carry out this exercise if you suffer from high blood pressure or other cardiovascular problems, have diabetes, are pregnant or have serious health issues. If in doubt you should always consult your doctor.) As with all breathing exercises, you should not carry out the nose-freeing exercise directly after eating.

1. Take a small, calm breath in through the nose and a small, calm breath out through the nose.

2.   Hold your nose closed with your fingers, in order to keep in the air.

3.   Walk as many steps as you can, while holding your breath. Try to build up a middle to strong air shortage, without overdoing it.

4.   When you start breathing again, just breathe through the nose. Try to calm your breathing straight away.

5.   After you have started breathing again, your first breath will probably be stronger. Take care to calm your breath as quickly as possible, by suppressing your second and third breaths.

6.   You should be able to normalise your respiration within two or three breaths. If your breath is irregular or

heavier than usual, you will have held it for too long.

7. Wait 1 or 2 minutes before you repeat your breath-holding exercise.

8. In order to prepare for longer breath-holding, you should first take a few breaths, starting slowly and then increasing the speed every time.

9. Repeat the whole exercise for a total of 6 breaths, so that your need for air seems quite strong.

Generally, this exercise loosens the blockage in the nose, even if you are suffering from a head cold. As soon as the benefit of the breath-holding exercise starts to weaken, the nose will probably start to feel blocked again. You will notice an improvement in the results as you increase the number of steps you take while holding your breath. When you can take a total of 80 steps, your nose should remain unblocked. 80 steps is really a realistic target and you can expect to increase the number by about 10 steps per week.

If you suffer regularly from a nose blockage, it should become easier to breathe through the nose again, very soon. You will no longer need any prescription-free decongestants, anti-histamines or cortisone nose sprays! When you hold your breath, you greatly increase the concentration of Nitrogen Monoxide in your nasal cavity, which results in expansion of the nasal passages and in gentle and light nose-breathing. When you do the breath-holding exercises later on in the book, you will notice that your ability to hold your breath improves, which will lead to more nasal freedom.

Through consistent nose-breathing and practising the above exercise, you can keep your nose free, even if you have a cold.

Light breathing as the key to success.

Ideal Respiration

Authentic teachers of Indian yoga and traditional Chinese medicine have long promoted the philosophy of effortless breathing. I use the word "authentic" to describe practitioners who have a profound knowledge about breathing and how it effects the physiology, as opposed to those who do not. Many modern yoga teachers instruct their students to breathe deeply, to remove poisons out of the body. Authentic teachers know that less is more, when it comes to breathing. The traditional Chinese philosophy of Taoism describes ideal breathing appropriately as "so soft, that the fine hairs in the nostrils do not move". Real health and inner peace result from peaceful breathing through the nose into the abdomen, which is effortless, soft and rhythmical and which pauses gently before exhaling. This is how humans breathed naturally before modern life changed everything.

What is a Deep Breath? Uncovering the Myth

Sometimes, the same word has different meanings for different people. Take the word "deep" as an example. "Deep" can be interpreted as "a long way from the top". But this is a little ambiguous. The floor of the deep end of a swimming pool is obviously further away from the surface than the floor of the shallow end, but when we use the word "deep" with reference to taking a deep breath, it can be interpreted in many ways.

This instruction is often given by stress counsellors, yoga practitioners and sport trainers, leading to the student taking a big breath into the lungs, often with an open mouth, while activating the upper chest. This kind of breathing is big, but flat and not deep. It is completely wrong if you want to achieve an increased circulation of Oxygen to the whole body.

If we use the definition "far from the top" in the context of deep breathing, we are referring to the "top" as the top of the lungs or upper chest. A deep breath means breathing into the deepest part of the lungs. This means using the main breathing muscle, the diaphragm, which separates the chest from the abdomen. During quiet times, healthy animals and babies breathe deeply and quietly. Every time you inhale, the abdomen stretches gently outwards and it retracts with every exhale. There is no need for strain; breathing continues silently and regularly and, more importantly, through the nose. If you want to learn about good breathing, watch a baby or a healthy pet, whose breathing has not yet been impacted by the modern lifestyle.

The Diaphragm

The diaphragm is dome-shaped muscle tissue that separates the thorax (which hosts the heart and the lungs) from the abdomen (which hosts the intestines, stomach, liver and kidneys). The diaphragm serves as our main breathing muscle and ensures deep and efficient breathing, if used properly. Bad breathing habits do not use the diaphragm fully and cause inefficient over-breathing from the upper chest.

Abdomen respiration is more efficient, even due to the form of the lungs. As they are narrow at the top and wider at the bottom the circulation of blood is greater in the lower lobe than it is in the upper lobe. Fast breathing into the chest does not use the lower part of the lung, which can influence the amount of Oxygen being transported through the blood and can, in turn, lead to a greater CO_2 reduction. In addition, breathing in the upper chest activates the fight or flight reaction which increases stress and makes breathing harder.

Watch your own respiration when you are stressed or watch the breathing of nervous relatives, friends or colleagues – you will see that this type of respiration happens mostly in the chest and is at a higher than normal rate. When we are stressed, we tend to over-breathe and fall back on mouth-breathing. Stressed breathing is quicker than normal, is audible and causes visible movement. You may also often hear sighs.

Many people breathe like this all the time, every minute of every day. They find themselves in a fight or flight condition with a high adrenalin level.

Even the best stress counsellors, psychologists or psychotherapists would not be able to start helping their patients if they have not tackled their dysfunctional breathing first. If Oxygen to the brain has been reduced, no argumentation or discussion can correct the situation. Stressed and frightened patients can only make progress when they tackle their bad breathing habits.

On the other side, healthy people who are relaxed and relatively stress-free use abdomen respiration: Slowly, softly, calmly, regularly, hardly noticeably, silently and through the nose. In order to achieve this kind of breathing and to reduce the negative effects of over-breathing, it is important to activate the parasympathetic nervous system of the body to create the relaxation. You must adjust your breathing habits to be able to use your diaphragm properly. Avoid sighs, panting and breathing through the mouth. Get used to breathing slowly, softly, calmly and quietly in a relaxed manner through the nose. This is how we should breathe all the time when in a resting state, every minute of every day.

Within a very short time you will notice that you are more peaceful and energetic and can sleep better. The positive effect of abdomen respiration will change every aspect of your health, including your sporting performance. An additional advantage is that it supports lymphatic drainage. The lymphatic system is basically your own drainage system which conducts waste materials and surplus fluid out of the body. As the lymphatic system does not have a heart, it relies on movement of the muscles, including the diaphragm, to pump waste out of the body.

During abdomen respiration, the lymph glands draw, neutralise and destroy dead cells, reduce the collection of fluids and improve the detoxification of the body. The natural advantage of abdomen respiration is that it improves the quality of the blood flow, increases the supply of Oxygen to the working muscles and reduces the symptoms of fear, which are associated with over-breathing. If you return to the natural and efficient breathing habits with which you are born, you can enjoy better health and maximise your sports or training performance. Use the following exercise to help you to perform abdomen respiration during resting times and sport until it becomes routine again.

Exercise 2: Breathe in lightly to breathe properly

During the breathing process, Oxygen is drawn into the lungs and superfluous Carbon Dioxide is exhaled. The breathing centre of the brain is continuously watching the PH, Carbon Dioxide and, to a lesser extent, the Oxygen values. If the Carbon Dioxide in the blood sinks below its pre-set level, the breathing centre sends an impulse which tells the breathing muscles that it should breathe in order to release the superfluous gas. If we are talking about breathing too much over a period of a few hours up to days, as during chronic stress, the breathing centre regulates less tolerance to Carbon Dioxide. A below average tolerance to Carbon Dioxide leads to the breathing centre increasing the rate that it sends the impulses to the breathing muscles which, in turn, results in over-breathing in general and breathlessness during physical activity.

You are carrying out the exercise correctly when you slow down and reduce your respiration in order to create a tolerable air requirement. Air requirement means an accumulation of arterial Carbon Dioxide, which has the aim of resetting the tolerance of the breathing centre to this gas. To support that, it is helpful to practise pressing lightly on the chest and abdomen. Try to maintain your air requirement over a period of 4 to 5 minutes. It is useful to sit in front of a mirror while doing this exercise, in order to watch your breath movements.

1. Sit up straight. Relax your shoulders. Imagine there is a piece of string attached to the top of your head, gently stretching the back of your

head upwards. Feel how the space between your ribs begins to widen.

2. Lay one hand on your chest and one directly over your navel.

3. Feel how your abdomen moves gently outwards while inhaling and inwards while exhaling.

4. As you breathe, press gently on the chest and abdomen, causing resistance to the movement.

5. Breathe against the hands and concentrate on reducing the size of every single breath.

6. Draw less air with every breath than you would like to. Make your breath smaller or shorter.

7. Gently slow down and reduce your breathing movement until you feel a tolerable need for air.

8. Breathe out in a relaxed way. Let the natural elasticity of your lungs and diaphragm do their job with every exhalation. Imagine a balloon which slowly and gently deflates all by itself.

9. When your breaths become smaller and exhaling becomes more relaxed, you will notice a reduction in breath movement. Perhaps you can see it in the mirror.

With a simple exercise like this, you can reduce your breathing movements by 20 to 30 percent. If your abdomen muscles contract, twitch or tense up, or your breathing rhythm becomes irregular and out of control, the air deficiency is too great. Stop the exercise for about 15 seconds and then start again when the air deficiency has been overcome.

At first you can probably only keep the deficiency up for 20 seconds before the urge to breathe becomes too strong. With a little practice you will be able to extend the time of air deficiency. Remember, you are trying to create an air deficiency which is tolerable but not stressful. Try to maintain a tolerable need for air for about 3 to 5 minutes each time.

Carry out the exercise in sets of 2, each for 5 minutes. This should be enough to help you to reset your breathing centre and improve your body's tolerance to Carbon Dioxide. Carrying out this exercise increases the collection of Carbon Dioxide in the blood which causes specific physiological changes to the body. These include:

- A feeling of increased warmth arising from the widening of the blood vessels.

- A light pink colour in the face.

- Increased production of watery saliva in the mouth which is a sign that your body is in a relaxed mode and the parasympathetic nervous system is activated.

All these changes are normal and should not cause any discomfort. If you become dizzy or experience fear during a breathing exercise, it is better to cease the exercise and consult an expert, who can tell you if you are doing the exercise correctly.

Reduce Injuries and Fatigue

Most physicians recommend physical exercise for good health. This begs the question: When does exercise become harmful? More importantly, what can we do to enjoy the advantages of physical exercise without endangering our health? The key to the answer lies in the control of stress which the body endures during training – more precisely, oxidative stress which is caused by too many free radicals which are spread throughout our system.

Free radicals are molecules which are created from Oxygen during metabolic activity. We all produce a certain number of free radicals during respiration. Normal values do not cause a problem because the resistance mechanism in your body is capable of neutralising them with antioxidants, such as glutathione, ubiquinone, flavonoids and vitamins A, E and C. However, when our resistance is overwhelmed by too many free radicals, it can cause damage to the cells and affect our health.

This is known as oxidative stress. Free radicals are extremely reactive and attack our cells, leading to tissue damage and negatively influencing lipids, proteins and DNA. We produce more free radicals than normal during physical activity because of the increase in respiration and metabolism. This leads to an imbalance between the production of free radicals and the anti-oxidants which are necessary for detoxification. This, in turn, leads to muscle weakness, tiredness and over-training.

Studies into body training, regular endurance sport, marathons and extreme competitions have consistently found that the number of antioxidants increased after intensive physical exercise or extreme competitions, while the production of free radicals rose.

Sportsmen are often ordered to take regular large doses of antioxidants to eliminate any potential imbalance between antioxidants and free radicals. It may seem good advice at first sight, but studies about the use of dietary antioxidants for reducing oxidative stress and muscle injuries caused by exercise have, up to now, led to mixed results.

An alternative and completely natural method to protect from the excessive accumulation of free radicals, is to supplement regular training with breath-holding exercises. This method is inexpensive, non-toxic, less controversial than dietary supplements and offers effective protection against oxidative stress. Breath-holding after exhalation leads to a reduction in

Oxygen saturation and an increase in lactic acid. At the same time the Carbon Dioxide level rises, leading to an increase in the concentration of Hydrogen ions which acidify the blood.

Repeated implementation of breathing pauses offsets the effect of the lactic acid and causes the body to make adjustments, in order to delay acidosis (increased acid in the blood) so that the sportsman can continue without the tiredness he had been experiencing. Research has shown that breath-holding exercises can improve the tolerance of an individual to hypoxemia (low Oxygen content in the blood), lower the acidity of the blood by removing oxidative stress and reducing the build-up of lactic acid.

Blood acidosis and oxidative stress have been significantly reduced in athletes with many years of respiration training, such as divers. This suggests that extensive implementation of breath-training can prevent the negative effects of exercise-related free radicals.

Research over a period of thirty years has examined the mitigating factors of movement-induced oxidative stress, where the type of activity, duration, intensity and ability of the individual were all taken into consideration. The right dosage of physical exercise varied, of course, from person to person, depending on their physical condition and training habits, but the results of numerous studies show that oxidative stress can be avoided best through regular exercise in combination with breath-training.

The body is very good at adapting to regular physical activity but can not always react quickly enough to protect itself from the sudden ingress of free radicals which occurs during high-intensity training.

The best way to cut down the oxidative stress and to increase the natural anti-oxidative resistance in your body is to train several times a week with a measured, pleasant intensity from which you can easily recover.

If you are a recreational sportsman who does little or no sport during the week, but who trains intensively at the weekend, it will probably cause more harm than benefit.

Breathing exercises during sport to improve physical performance.

Breathing Exercise during Exertion

During the times when you feel like deviating from your normal breathing technique, you increase the danger of breathing badly. This is particularly the case during physical exertion when the body demands more Oxygen in order to supply the muscles with energy. Breathing becomes quicker but the supply of Oxygen does not necessarily improve. You have learned how to breathe effectively and you know what you need to take into consideration in order to improve your Oxygen supply. I will now show you two exercises to help you maintain an ideal breathing technique, even during periods of excessive exertion.

Exercise 3: Breath Regeneration, Improved Concentration

Carry out this exercise for 3 to 5 minutes when you need to recuperate from physical activity and calm your breathing:

1. Breathe out as usual through the nose.

2. Pinch your nose for 2 to 5 seconds in order to hold your breath.

3. Breathe for 10 seconds normally through the nose.

4. Repeat the first three steps

With this simple exercise you can return your Oxygen and Carbon Dioxide balance to normal levels. At the same time, you will increase your lung volume which will, in turn, improve sustainably your absorption capacity of Oxygen into the blood.

Exercise 4: Simulate Altitude Training: Bike Riding, Running, Swimming

The following exercise is meant for active sportsmen during training. Normally, in altitude training the body modifies itself to cope with the decreased Oxygen supply in the air by increasing the production of red blood corpuscles (erythropoiesis). This increases your capacity to take in Oxygen and to transport it around the body. This effect does not take place for some time. You must, therefore, carry out the exercise continuously and consistently in order to maintain a positive effect. In addition, it offers great benefits for your body and health if you regularly and conscientiously implement it.

- After running for 10 to 15 minutes, exhale gently and hold your breath until you feel a strong air deficiency.

The length of the breath-hold should be between 10 and 40 steps, depending on your running pace.

- After holding your breath jog for about a minute, breathing through your nose, until you have partly regained your breath.

- Repeat the breath-hold 8 to 10 times during your run. The breath-hold should be a challenge and your breathing should normalise within a few breaths.

Let this simple exercise become part of your training routine, the effects will be increasingly noticeable.

Breathing Exercise for Relaxation

Why breathing is so Important for Relaxation during Rest Periods.

Deliberate breathing helps you to relax in every-day life. Your body can only come to rest and power down when your Oxygen supply is ideal and your body has found a balance between Oxygen and Carbon Dioxide. This is absolutely necessary to help your mind relax and become peaceful. You already know that deep breathing is decisive in reducing your respiratory movements and with it the movement of your whole body as much as possible. This is how to achieve deep calm. What you should be paying attention to in your every-day life should be followed even more intensively here to help your body reduce its stress level even more. The following exercise should help you to achieve that.

Exercise 5: The Relaxation Ritual

1. Sit up straight so as to give your lungs enough room.

2. Close your ears with your index finger

3. Inhale slowly and consciously through the nose and count to eight.

4. Hold your breath and count to four

5. Exhale through the nose, creating a clear humming tone, while counting to eight.

6. Before you repeat Point 3, wait a few seconds to increase your Oxygen demand.

7. Repeat this exercise ten times

8.   Take care to keep the rhythm even
     and low. Do not breathe too quickly
     but do not become breathless.

With conscious and slow breathing, together
with the increase in Carbon Monoxide
absorption, after ten repeats you should notice
an appreciable easing of tension. When you feel
that the effect is wearing off, after a short time
you can repeat it to regain your relaxation status.

Concluding Remarks

When deciding whether or not to make lifestyle changes, it is important to consider the individual's health. Taking a look at your lifestyle is useful in order to adapt your exercises so that they cause the least disruption to your working time and present training schedules. I can understand that it is a challenge to find time to carry out exercises in stressful times. This is why this book offers you quick, simple and achievable techniques which can fit into any current routine.

There is no doubt that bad breathing techniques can lead to fatigue, loss of concentration and poor productivity. If you can spare only half an hour per day to carry out these exercises, your energy level, well-being and your performance will rise. I have seen hundreds of people who have benefited from investing a small amount of time to improve the Oxygen supply to their bodies.

The best way to approach the techniques in this book is to regard this as a change of lifestyle and something that can be integrated into your life, not as a list of exercises that must be carried out formally all day long. This way they will become a part of your daily routine and will not be seen as a task or obligation.

This way, you achieve, with just a little commitment, a huge and sustainable effect. When you have achieved lasting, optimal respiration, you optimise your Oxygen supply, your Carbon Dioxide balance and your Nitrogen Oxide values. Without additional training you can increase your physical performance capacity and your physical and psychological health. When your body is in balance and functions with less stress, your mind will be more relaxed and peaceful, something which you can benefit from every day. The only thing you need to do is carry out a few exercises and, above all, be aware of your breathing technique.

Thank you for taking the time to read this book. I wish you much success and gentle breathing!

Did you enjoy my book?

Now you have read my book, you know how best to optimize your breathing. This is why I am asking you now for a small favour. Customer reviews are an important part of every product offered by Amazon. It is the first thing that customers look at and, more often than not, is the main reason whether or not they decide to buy the product. Considering the endless number of products available at Amazon, this factor is becoming increasingly important.

If you liked my book, I would be more than grateful if you could leave your review by Amazon. How do you do that? Just click on the "Write a customer review"-button (as shown below), which you find on the Amazon product page of my book or your orders site:

Review this product

Share your thoughts with other customers

Write a customer review

Just write a short review as to whether you particularly liked my book or what you gained from reading it. It will not take more than a few minutes, honestly!

Be assured, I will read every review personally. It will help me a lot to improve my books and to tailor them to your wishes.

For this I say to you:

Thank you very much!

Yours

Lutz

List of references

Barczok, Michael (2018)

Luft nach oben: wie richtiges Atmen uns stärker macht

Krawietz-Bispinck, Veronika (1992)

Ganzheitlich beten: Körpersprache, Atemtechnik, Rosenkranz

Hauk, Andrea

Biologie in unserer Zeit (01.06.2017)

Putzwahn und Atemtechnik

Krusche, Gustav (1906)

Das Atmen beim Sprechen, Lesen und Singen: ein Beitrag zu dessen Beachtung, Regelung und Übung

Boren, Mark (2008)

Musik atmen: eine Richtlinie für Bläser und
Sänger

McKeown, Patrick (2018)
Erfolgsfaktor Sauerstoff: Wissenschaftlich
belegte Atemtechniken, um die Gesundheit zu
verbessern und die sportliche Leistung zu
steigern

Kaminoff, Leslie Kaminoff, Leslie, Matthews
(2013)
Yoga-Anatomie: Ihr Begleiter durch die Asanas,
Bewegungen und Atemtechniken

Proctor, Donald F (1980)
Breathing, speech and song

Bormann, Julia
Sport Praxis (2017)
Entspannungsübungen: Ausgleich für
Alltagsstress

Döbele, Martina

Heilberufe (01.09.2014)

Richtig durchatmen: Pneumonieprophylaxe

Fessler, Norbert Knoll, Michaela

Praxis der Psychomotorik (2012)

Kinder stark machen: Basics zur Atemschulung

Anthony Anhold (2013)

The Breathing Exercise Bible: Relaxation and Meditation

Techniques for Happiness and Healthy Living

Richard Brennan (2018)

How to Breathe: Improve Your Breathing for Health, Happiness and Well-Being (Includes over 30 Breathing Exercises and Techniques)

Disclaimer

©2019, Lutz Schneider

1st Edition

Made in the USA
Monee, IL
29 January 2025

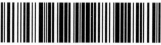

11217945R00065